The Effortless Mediterranean Recipe Collection

An Essential and Complete Guide For Homemade cooking

Alison Russell

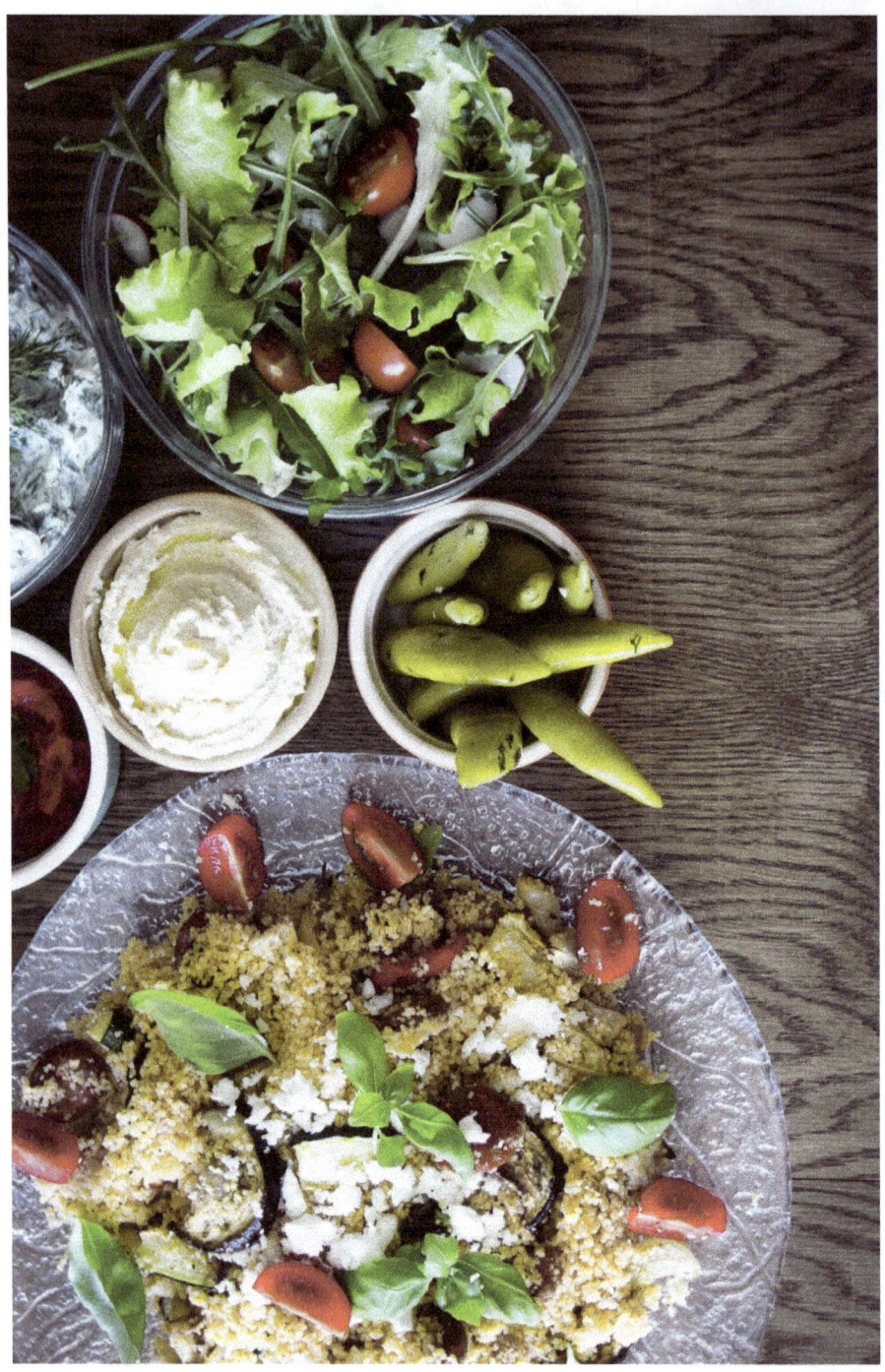

© **Copyright 2020 - All rights reserved.**

The content contained within this book may not be reproduced, duplicated or transmitted without direct written permission from the author or the publisher.

Under no circumstances will any blame or legal responsibility be held against the publisher, or author, for any damages, reparation, or monetary loss due to the information contained within this book. Either directly or indirectly.

Legal Notice:

This book is copyright protected. This book is only for personal use. You cannot amend, distribute, sell, use, quote or paraphrase any part, or the content within this book, without the consent of the author or publisher.

Disclaimer Notice:

Please note the information contained within this document is for educational and entertainment purposes only. All effort has been executed to present accurate, up to date, and reliable, complete information. No warranties of any kind are declared or implied. Readers acknowledge that the author is not engaging in the rendering of legal, financial, medical or professional advice. The content within this book has been derived from various sources. Please consult a licensed professional before attempting any techniques outlined in this book.

By reading this document, the reader agrees that under no circumstances is the author responsible for any losses, direct or indirect, which are incurred as a result of the use of information contained within this document, Including, but not limited to, — errors, omissions, or inaccuracies.

Table of contents

Breakfast 9
    Mediterranean Smoothie 11
    Fruit Smoothie 12
    Strawberry-Rhubarb Smoothie 15
    Chia-Pomegranate Smoothie 17
    Tomato and Zucchini Frittata 18
    Smoked Salmon Scramble 21
Lunch 23
    Vegetable and Red Lentil Stew 25
    Roasted Vegetables 28
    Ratatouille 30
    Sautéed Green Beans with Tomatoes 32
    Baked Tomatoes and Chickpeas 35
    Creamy Cauliflower Chickpea Curry 37
    Cauliflower Rice Risotto with Mushrooms 39
    Sweet Potato Chickpea Buddha Bowl 42
    Zucchini Patties 44
    Zucchini Crisp 46

Creamy Sweet Potatoes and Collards 48

Shrimp and Spaghetti Squash Bowls 50

Scallop Teriyaki 53

Shrimp and Tomato Creole 55

Mahi-Mahi and Tomato Bowls 57

Alfredo Tuscan Shrimp with Penne 59

Tuna with Shirataki Noodles 61

Grits with Shrimp 62

Basil Pesto 64

Creamy Cider Yogurt Dressing 67

Basic French Vinaigrette 68

Mediterranean Lamb Bowl 69

Lamb Burger 72

Quick Herbed Lamb and Pasta 74

Marinated Lamb Kebabs with Crunchy Yogurt Dressing 76

Garlic Pork Tenderloin and Lemony Orzo 79

Roasted Pork with Apple-Dijon Sauce 81

Pressure Cooker Moroccan Pot Roast 83

Shawarma Pork Tenderloin with Pitas 86

Desserts 90

Honey Almonds 92

Chocolate-Dipped Citrus Fruit..95

Banana-Cinnamon "Ice Cream "..97

Sweet Peach Jam 98

Pear Sauce 99

Brownie Muffins.. 101

French Toast Bites...103

Cinnamon Sugar Roasted Chickpeas....................................104

Glazed Pears with Hazelnuts 105

Lemony Blackberry Granita...107

Breakfast

Mediterranean Smoothie

Preparation Time: 5 minutes

Cooking Time: 5 minutes

Servings: 2

Ingredients:

- 2 cups of baby spinach
- 1 teaspoon fresh ginger root
- 1 frozen banana, pre-sliced
- 1 small mango
- ½ cup beet juice
- ½ cup of skim milk
- 4-6 ice cubes

Directions:

1. Take all ingredients and place them in your blender. Blend together until thick and smooth. Serve.

Nutrition:

Calories: 168

Protein: 4 g

Fat: 1 g

Carbohydrates: 39 g

Fruit Smoothie

Preparation Time: 5 minutes

Cooking Time: 0 minutes

Servings: 2

Ingredients:

- 2 cups blueberries (or any fresh or frozen fruit, cut into pieces if the fruit is large)
- 2 cups unsweetened almond milk
- 1 cup crushed ice
- ½ teaspoon ground ginger (or other dried ground spice such as turmeric, cinnamon, or nutmeg)

Directions:

1. In a blender, combine the blueberries, almond milk, ice, and ginger. Blend until smooth.

Nutrition:

Calories: 125

Protein: 2g

Carbohydrates: 23g

Fat: 4g

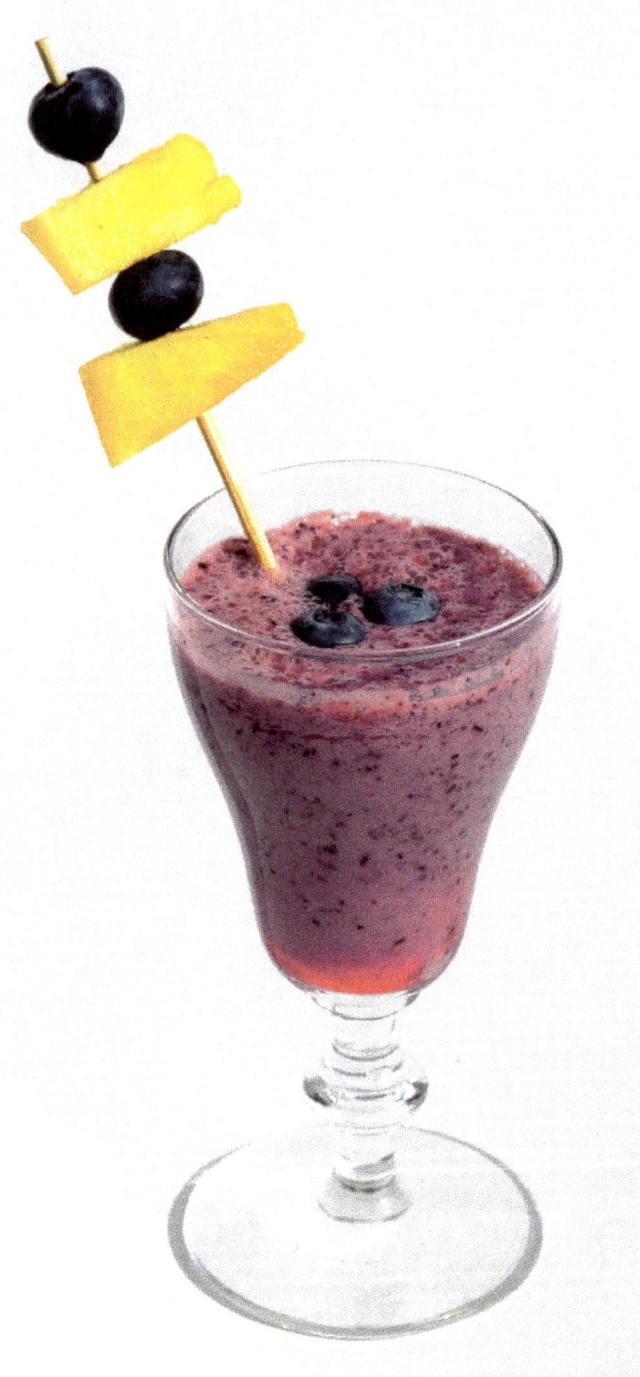

Strawberry-Rhubarb Smoothie

Preparation Time: 5 minutes

Cooking Time: 3 minutes

Servings: 1

Ingredients:

- 1 rhubarb stalk, chopped
- 1 cup sliced fresh strawberries
- ½ cup plain Greek yogurt
- 2 tablespoons honey
- Pinch ground cinnamon
- 3 ice cubes

Directions:

Place a small saucepan filled with water over high heat and bring to a boil. Add the rhubarb and boil for 3 minutes. Drain and transfer the rhubarb to a blender.

Add the strawberries, yogurt, honey, and cinnamon and pulse the mixture until it is smooth. Add the ice and blend until thick, with no ice lumps remaining. Pour the smoothie into a glass and enjoy cold.

Nutrition:

Calories: 295

Fat: 8g

Carbohydrates: 56g

Protein: 6g

Chia-Pomegranate Smoothie

Preparation Time: 5 minutes

Cooking Time: 0 minutes

Servings: 2

Ingredients:

- 1 cup pure pomegranate juice (no sugar added)
- 1 cup frozen berries
- 1 cup coarsely chopped kale
- 2 tablespoons chia seeds
- 3 Medjool dates, pitted and coarsely chopped
- Pinch ground cinnamon

Directions:

1. In a blender, combine the pomegranate juice, berries, kale, chia seeds, dates, and cinnamon and pulse until smooth. Pour into glasses and serve.

Nutrition:

Calories: 275

Fat: 5g

Carbohydrates: 59g

Protein: 5g

Tomato and Zucchini Frittata

Preparation Time: 10 minutes

Cooking Time: 18 minutes

Servings: 4

Ingredients:

- 3 eggs
- 3 egg whites
- 1/2 cup unsweetened almond milk
- 1/2 teaspoon sea salt
- 1/8 teaspoon freshly ground black pepper
- 2 tablespoons extra-virgin olive oil
- 1 zucchini, chopped
- 8 cherry tomatoes, halved
- 1/4 cup (about 2 ounces) grated Parmesan cheese

Directions:

1. Heat the oven's broiler to high, adjusting the oven rack to the center position.
2. Whip the eggs, egg whites, almond milk, sea salt, and pepper. Set aside.
3. Heat the olive oil until it shimmers.
4. Attach the zucchini and tomatoes and cook for 5 minutes, stirring occasionally.

5. Stream the egg mixture over the vegetables and cook for about 4 minutes without stirring until the eggs set around the edges.
6. Using a silicone spatula, pull the set eggs away from the edges of the pan. Lean the pan in all directions to allow the unset eggs to fill the spaces along the edges. Cook for about 4 minutes more without stirring until the edges set again.
7. Sprinkle the eggs with the Parmesan. Transfer the pan to the broiler. Dissolve the cheese melts and the eggs are puffy. Cut into wedges to serve.

Nutrition:

Calories: 223, Protein: 14g, Total Carbohydrates: 13g, Fiber: 4g, Sodium: 476mg

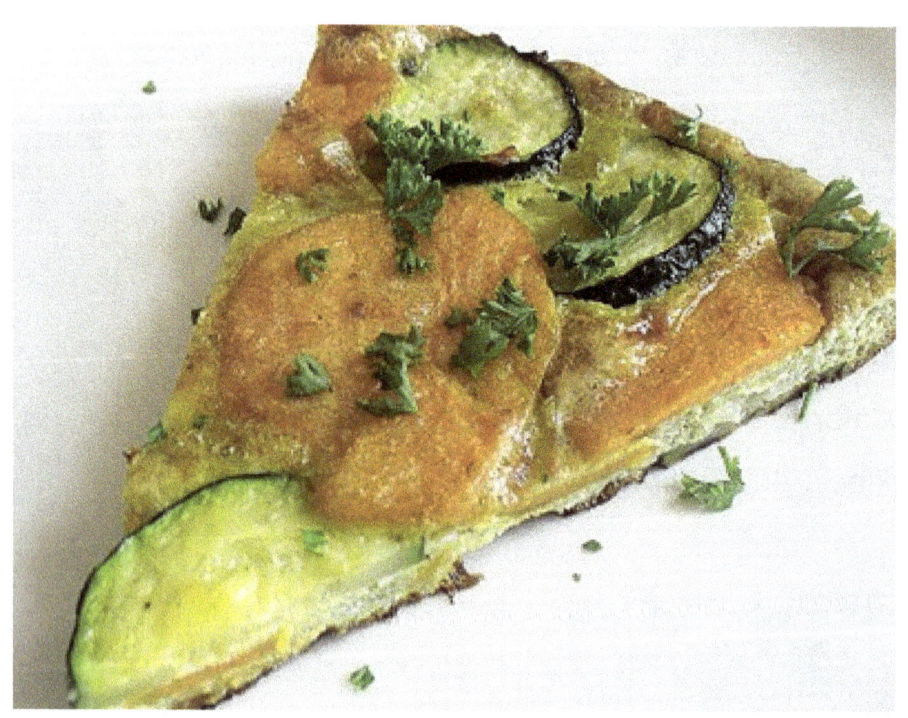

Smoked Salmon Scramble

Preparation Time: 5 minutes

Cooking Time: 10 minutes

Servings: 4

Ingredients:

- 4 eggs
- 6 egg whites
- 1/8 teaspoon freshly ground black pepper
- 2 tablespoons extra-virgin olive oil
- 1/2 red onion, finely chopped
- 4 ounces smoked salmon, flaked
- 2 tablespoons capers, drained

Directions:

1. Whip the eggs, egg whites, and pepper. Set aside.
2. Heat the olive oil until it shimmers.
3. Attach the red onion and cook for about 3 minutes, stirring occasionally, until soft.
4. Add the salmon and capers and cook for 1 minute.
5. Attach the egg mixture to the pan and cook for 3 to 5 minutes, stirring frequently, or until the eggs are set.

Nutrition:

Calories: 189

Protein: 16g

Total Carbohydrates: 2g

Fiber: 1g

Total Fat: 13g

Sodium: 806mg

Lunch

Vegetable and Red Lentil Stew

Prep time: 10 minutes | Cook time: 35 minutes | Serves 6

1 tablespoon extra-virgin olive oil

2 onions, peeled and finely diced

6½ cups water

2 zucchini, finely diced

4 celery stalks, finely diced

3 cups red lentils

1 teaspoon dried oregano

1 teaspoon salt, plus more as needed

1. **Heat the olive oil in a large pot over medium heat.**
2. **Add the onions and sauté for about 5 minutes, stirring constantly, or until the onions are softened.**
3. **Stir in the water, zucchini, celery, lentils, oregano, and salt and bring the mixture to a boil.**

4. **Reduce the heat to low and let simmer covered for 30 minutes, stirring occasionally, or until the lentils are tender.**
5. **Taste and adjust the seasoning as needed.**

Per Serving

calories: 387 | fat: 4.4g | protein: 24.0g | carbs: 63.7g | fiber: 11.7g | sodium: 418mg

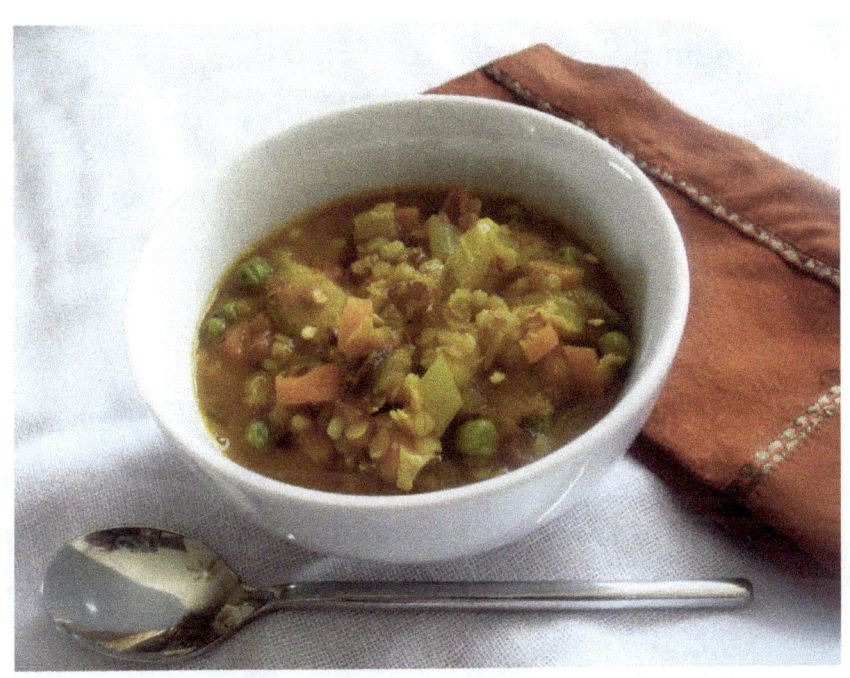

Roasted Vegetables

Prep time: 20 minutes | Cook time: 35 minutes | Serves 2

6 teaspoons extra-virgin olive oil, divided

2 cups fresh cauliflower florets

12 to 15 Brussels sprouts, halved

1 medium zucchini, cut into 1-inch rounds

1 medium sweet potato, peeled and cut into 2-inch cubes

1 red bell pepper, cut into 1-inch slices

Salt, to taste

1. **Preheat the oven to 425°F (220°C).**
2. **Add 2 teaspoons of olive oil, Brussels sprouts, sweet potato, and salt to a large bowl and toss until they are completely coated.**
3. **Transfer them to a large roasting pan and roast for 10 minutes, or until the Brussels sprouts are lightly browned.**
4. **Meantime, combine the cauliflower florets with 2 teaspoons of olive oil and salt in a separate bowl.**

5. Remove from the oven. Add the cauliflower florets to the roasting pan and roast for 10 minutes more.
6. Meanwhile, toss the zucchini and bell pepper with the remaining olive oil in a medium bowl until well coated. Season with salt.
7. Remove the roasting pan from the oven and stir in the zucchini and bell pepper. Continue roasting for 15 minutes, or until the vegetables are fork- tender.
8. Divide the roasted vegetables between two plates and serve warm.

Per Serving

calories: 333 | fat: 16.8g | protein: 12.2g | carbs: 37.6g | fiber: 11.0g | sodium: 329mg

Ratatouille

Prep time: 10 minutes | Cook time: 30 minutes | Serves 4

4 tablespoons extra-virgin olive oil, divided

1 cup diced zucchini

2 cups diced eggplant

1 cup diced onion

1 cup chopped green bell pepper

1 (15-ounce / 425-g) can no-salt-added diced tomatoes

½ teaspoon garlic powder

1 teaspoon ground thyme

Salt and freshly ground black pepper, to taste

1. **Heat 2 tablespoons of olive oil in a large saucepan over medium heat until it shimmers.**
2. **Add the zucchini and eggplant and sauté for 10 minutes, stirring occasionally. If necessary, add the remaining olive oil.**
3. **Stir in the onion and bell pepper and sauté for 5 minutes until softened.**
4. **Add the diced tomatoes with their juice, garlic powder, and thyme and stir to combine. Continue cooking for 15 minutes**

until the vegetables are cooked through, stirring occasionally. Sprinkle with salt and black pepper.

5. Remove from the heat and serve on a plate.

Per Serving

calories: 189 | fat: 13.7g | protein: 3.1g | carbs: 14.8g | fiber: 4.0g | sodium: 27mg

Sautéed Green Beans with Tomatoes

Prep time: 10 minutes | Cook time: 20 minutes | Serves 4

¼ cup extra-virgin olive oil

1 large onion, chopped

4 cloves garlic, finely chopped

1 pound (454 g) green beans, fresh or frozen, cut into 2-inch pieces

1½ teaspoons salt, divided

1 (15-ounce / 425-g) can diced tomatoes

½ teaspoon freshly ground black pepper

1. Heat the olive oil in a large skillet over medium heat.
2. Add the onion and garlic and sauté for 1 minute until fragrant.
3. Stir in the green beans and sauté for 3 minutes. Sprinkle with ½ teaspoon of salt.
4. Add the tomatoes, remaining salt, and pepper and stir to mix well. Cook for an additional 12 minutes, stirring occasionally, or until the green beans are crisp and tender.

5. Remove from the heat and serve warm.

Per Serving

calories: 219 | fat: 13.9g | protein: 4.0g | carbs: 17.7g | fiber: 6.2g | sodium: 843mg

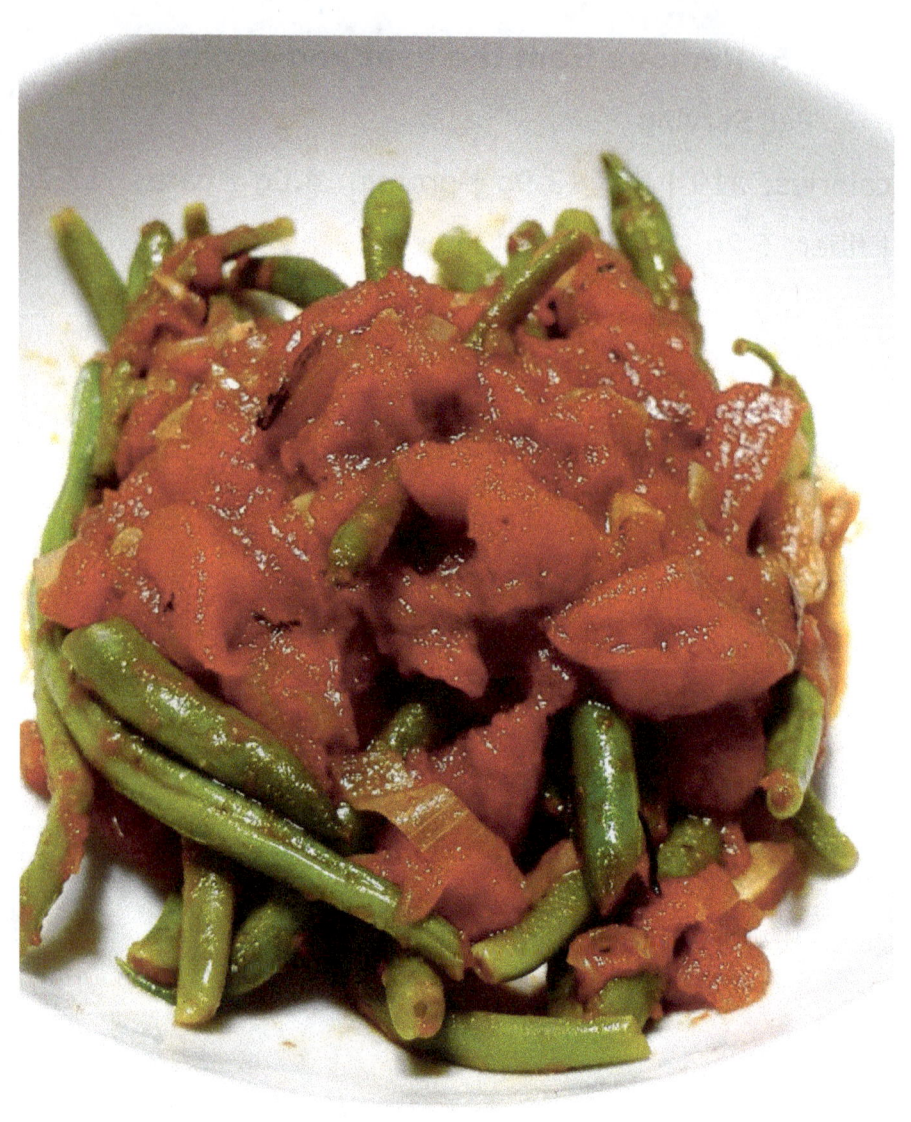

Baked Tomatoes and Chickpeas

Prep time: 15 minutes | Cook time: 40 to 45 minutes | Serves 4

1 tablespoon extra-virgin olive oil

½ medium onion, chopped

3 garlic cloves, chopped

¼ teaspoon ground cumin

2 teaspoons smoked paprika

2 (15-ounce / 425-g) cans chickpeas, drained and rinsed

4 cups halved cherry tomatoes

½ cup plain Greek yogurt, for serving

1 cup crumbled feta cheese, for serving

1. Preheat the oven to 425°F (220°C).
2. Heat the olive oil in an ovenproof skillet over medium heat.
3. Add the onion and garlic and sauté for about 5 minutes, stirring occasionally, or until tender and fragrant.
4. Add the paprika and cumin and cook for 2 minutes. Stir in the chickpeas and

tomatoes and allow to simmer for 5 to 10 minutes.
5. Transfer the skillet to the preheated oven and roast for 25 to 30 minutes, or until the mixture bubbles and thickens.
6. Remove from the oven and serve topped with yogurt and crumbled feta cheese.

Per Serving

calories: 411 | fat: 14.9g | protein: 20.2g | carbs: 50.7g | fiber: 13.3g | sodium: 443mg

Creamy Cauliflower Chickpea Curry

Prep time: 5 minutes | Cook time: 15 minutes | Serves 4

- 3 cups fresh or frozen cauliflower florets
- 2 cups unsweetened almond milk
- 1 (15-ounce / 425-g) can low-sodium chickpeas, drained and rinsed
- 1 tablespoon curry powder
- ¼ teaspoon garlic powder
- ¼ teaspoon ground ginger
- ⅛ teaspoon onion powder
- ¼ teaspoon salt
- 1 (15-ounce / 425-g) can coconut milk

1. Add the cauliflower florets, almond milk, chickpeas, coconut milk, curry powder, garlic powder, ginger, and onion powder to a large stockpot and stir to combine.

2. **Cover and cook over medium-high heat for 10 minutes, stirring occasionally.**
3. **Reduce the heat to low and continue cooking uncovered for 5 minutes, or until the cauliflower is tender.**
4. **Sprinkle with the salt and stir well. Serve warm.**

Per Serving

calories: 409 | fat: 29.6g | protein: 10.0g | carbs: 29.8g | fiber: 9.1g | sodium: 117mg

Cauliflower Rice Risotto with Mushrooms

Prep time: 5 minutes | Cook time: 10 minutes | Serves 4

1 teaspoon extra-virgin olive oil

½ cup chopped portobello mushrooms

4 cups cauliflower rice

½ cup plain Greek yogurt

¼ cup low-sodium vegetable broth

1 cup shredded Parmesan cheese

1. In a medium skillet, heat the olive oil over medium-low heat until shimmering.
2. Add the mushrooms and stir-fry for 3 minutes.
3. Stir in the cauliflower rice, yogurt, and vegetable broth. Cover and bring to a boil over high heat for 5 minutes, stirring occasionally.
4. Add the Parmesan cheese and stir to combine. Continue cooking for an

additional 3 minutes until the cheese is melted.

5. Divide the mixture into four bowls and serve warm.

Per Serving

calories: 167 | fat: 10.7g | protein: 12.1g | carbs: 8.1g | fiber: 3.0g | sodium: 326mg

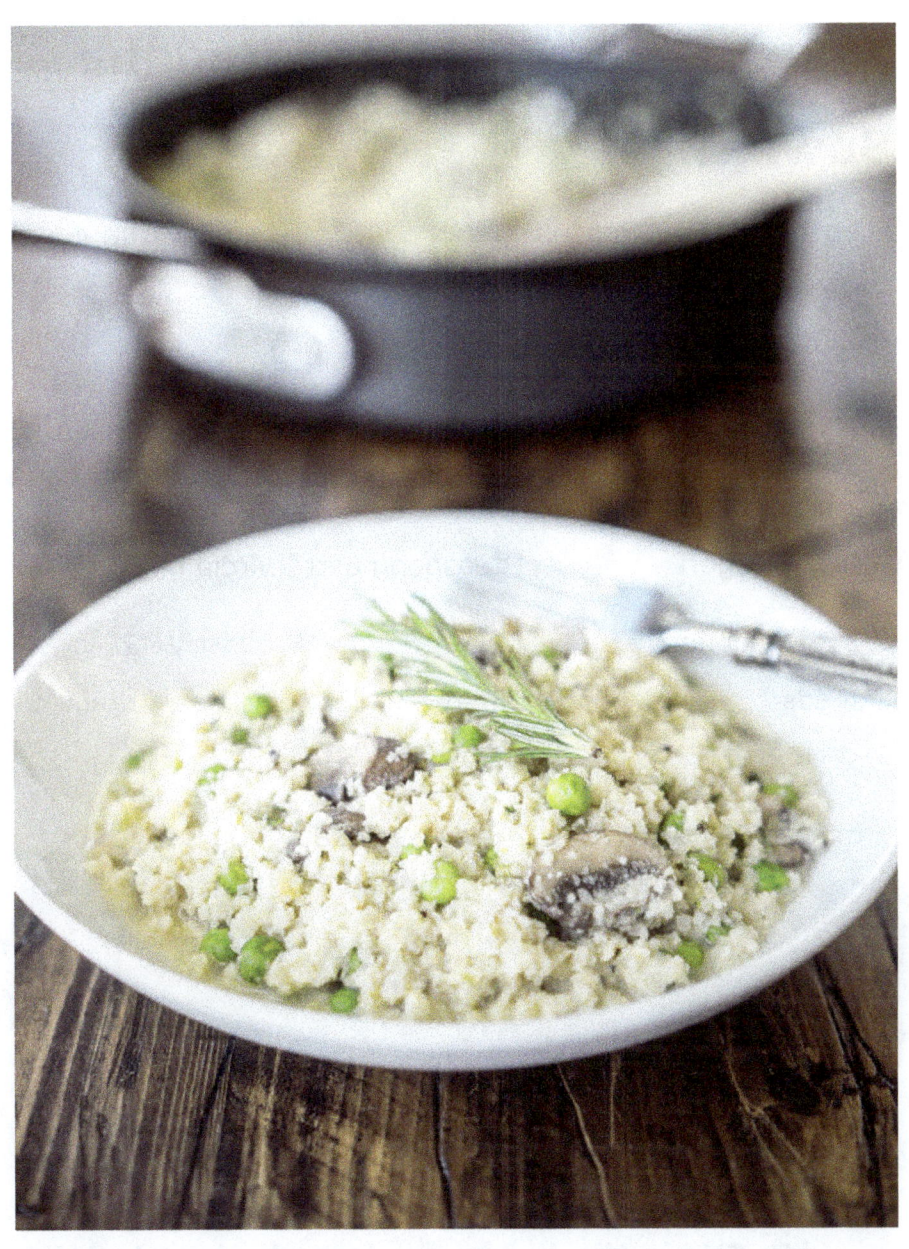

Sweet Potato Chickpea Buddha Bowl

Prep time: 10 minutes | Cook time: 10 to 15 minutes | Serves 2

Sauce:

1 tablespoon tahini

2 tablespoons plain Greek yogurt

2 tablespoons hemp seeds

1 garlic clove, minced Pinch salt

Freshly ground black pepper, to taste

Bowl:

1 small sweet potato, peeled and finely diced

1 teaspoon extra-virgin olive oil

1 cup from 1 (15-ounce / 425-g) can low-sodium chickpeas, drained and rinsed

2 cups baby kale

Make the Sauce

1. Whisk together the tahini and yogurt in a small bowl.
2. Stir in the hemp seeds and minced garlic. Season with salt pepper. Add 2 to 3

tablespoons water to create a creamy yet pourable consistency and set aside.

Make the Bowl

3. **Preheat the oven to 425ºF (220ºC). Line a baking sheet with parchment paper.**
4. **Place the sweet potato on the prepared baking sheet and drizzle with the olive oil. Toss well**
5. **Roast in the preheated oven for 10 to 15 minutes, stirring once during cooking, or until fork-tender and browned.**
6. **In each of 2 bowls, place ½ cup of chickpeas, 1 cup of baby kale, and half of the cooked sweet potato. Serve drizzled with half of the prepared sauce.**

Per Serving

calories: 323 | fat: 14.1g | protein: 17.0g | carbs: 36.0 g | fiber: 7.9g | sodium: 304mg

Zucchini Patties

Prep time: 15 minutes | Cook time: 5 minutes | Serves 2

- 2 medium zucchinis, shredded
- 1 teaspoon salt, divided
- 2 eggs
- 2 tablespoons chickpea flour
- 1 tablespoon chopped fresh mint
- 1 scallion, chopped
- 2 tablespoons extra-virgin olive oil

1. **Put the shredded zucchini in a fine-mesh strainer and season with ½ teaspoon of salt. Set aside.**
2. **Beat together the eggs, chickpea flour, mint, scallion, and remaining ½ teaspoon of salt in a medium bowl.**
3. **Squeeze the zucchini to drain as much liquid as possible. Add the zucchini to the egg mixture and stir until well incorporated.**
4. **Heat the olive oil in a large skillet over medium-high heat.**

5. **Drop the zucchini mixture by spoonfuls into the skillet. Gently flatten the zucchini with the back of a spatula.**
6. **Cook for 2 to 3 minutes or until golden brown. Flip and cook for an additional 2 minutes.**
7. **Remove from the heat and serve on a plate.**

Per Serving

calories: 264 | fat: 20.0g | protein: 9.8g | carbs: 16.1g | fiber: 4.0g | sodium: 1780mg

Zucchini Crisp

Prep time: 10 minutes | Cook time: 20 minutes | Serves 2

4 zucchinis, sliced into ½-inch rounds

½ cup unsweetened almond milk

1 teaspoon fresh lemon juice

1 teaspoon arrowroot powder

½ teaspoon salt, divided

½ cup whole wheat bread crumbs

¼ cup nutritional yeast

¼ cup hemp seeds

½ teaspoon garlic powder

¼ teaspoon crushed red pepper

¼ teaspoon black pepper

1. **Preheat the oven to 375°F (190°C). Line two baking sheets with parchment paper and set aside.**
2. **Put the zucchini in a medium bowl with the almond milk, lemon juice, arrowroot powder, and ¼ teaspoon of salt. Stir to mix well.**
3. **In a large bowl with a lid, thoroughly combine the bread crumbs, nutritional yeast, hemp seeds, garlic powder, crushed**

red pepper and black pepper. Add the zucchini in batches and shake until the slices are evenly coated.
4. Arrange the zucchini on the prepared baking sheets in a single layer.
5. Bake in the preheated oven for about 20 minutes, or until the zucchini slices are golden brown.
6. Season with the remaining ¼ teaspoon of salt before serving.

Per Serving

calories: 255 | fat: 11.3g | protein: 8.6g | carbs: 31.9g | fiber: 3.8g | sodium: 826mg

Creamy Sweet Potatoes and Collards

Prep time: 20 minutes | Cook time: 35 minutes | Serves 2

1 tablespoon avocado oil

3 garlic cloves, chopped

1 yellow onion, diced

½ teaspoon crushed red pepper flakes

1 large sweet potato, peeled and diced

2 bunches collard greens (about 2 pounds/907 g), stemmed, leaves chopped int 1-inch squares

1 (14.5-ounce / 411-g) can diced tomatoes with juice

1 (15-ounce / 425-g) can red kidney beans or chickpeas, drained and rinsed

1½ cups water

½ cup unsweetened coconut milk

Salt and black pepper, to taste

1. **In a large, deep skillet over medium heat, melt the avocado oil.**

2. Add the garlic, onion, and red pepper flakes and cook for 3 minutes. Stir in the sweet potato and collards.
3. Add the tomatoes with their juice, beans, water, and coconut milk and mix well. Bring the mixture just to a boil.
4. Reduce the heat to medium-low, cover, and simmer for about 30 minutes, or until softened.
5. Season to taste with salt and pepper and serve.

Per Serving

calories: 445 | fat: 9.6g | protein: 18.1g | carbs: 73.1g | fiber: 22.1g | sodium: 703mg

Shrimp and Spaghetti Squash Bowls

Prep time: 5 minutes | Cook time: 25 minutes | Serves 4

½ cup dry white wine
¼ teaspoon crushed red pepper flakes
1 large shallot, finely chopped
1 pound (454 g) jumbo shrimp, peeled and deveined
1 (28-ounce / 794-g) can crushed tomatoes
2 cloves garlic, minced
2½ pounds (1.1 kg) spaghetti squash
1 teaspoon olive oil
Salt and pepper, to taste
Parsley leaves (garnish)

1. At first, sprinkle some salt and pepper over the shrimp and keep them in a refrigerator until further use.

2. Hit the Sauté function on your Instant Pot, then add the olive oil and red pepper flakes into it. Sauté for 1 minute.
3. Add the shallot and cook for 3 minutes. Then add the garlic, cook for 1 minute.
4. Add the dry wine, tomatoes, and whole spaghetti squash in the pot. Select Manual settings with medium pressure for 20 minutes.
5. After the beep, do a Natural release. Remove the lid and the spaghetti squash.
6. Cut squash in half, remove its seed and stab with a fork to form spaghetti strands out of it. Keep them aside.
7. Select the Sauté function on your instant pot again, stir in shrimp.
8. Mix well the shrimp with sauce.
9. To serve, top the spaghetti squash with shrimp and sauce. Garnish it with parsley.

Per Serving

calories: 222 | fat: 4.4g | protein: 19.3g | carbs: 30.1g | fiber: 8.5g | sodium: 974mg

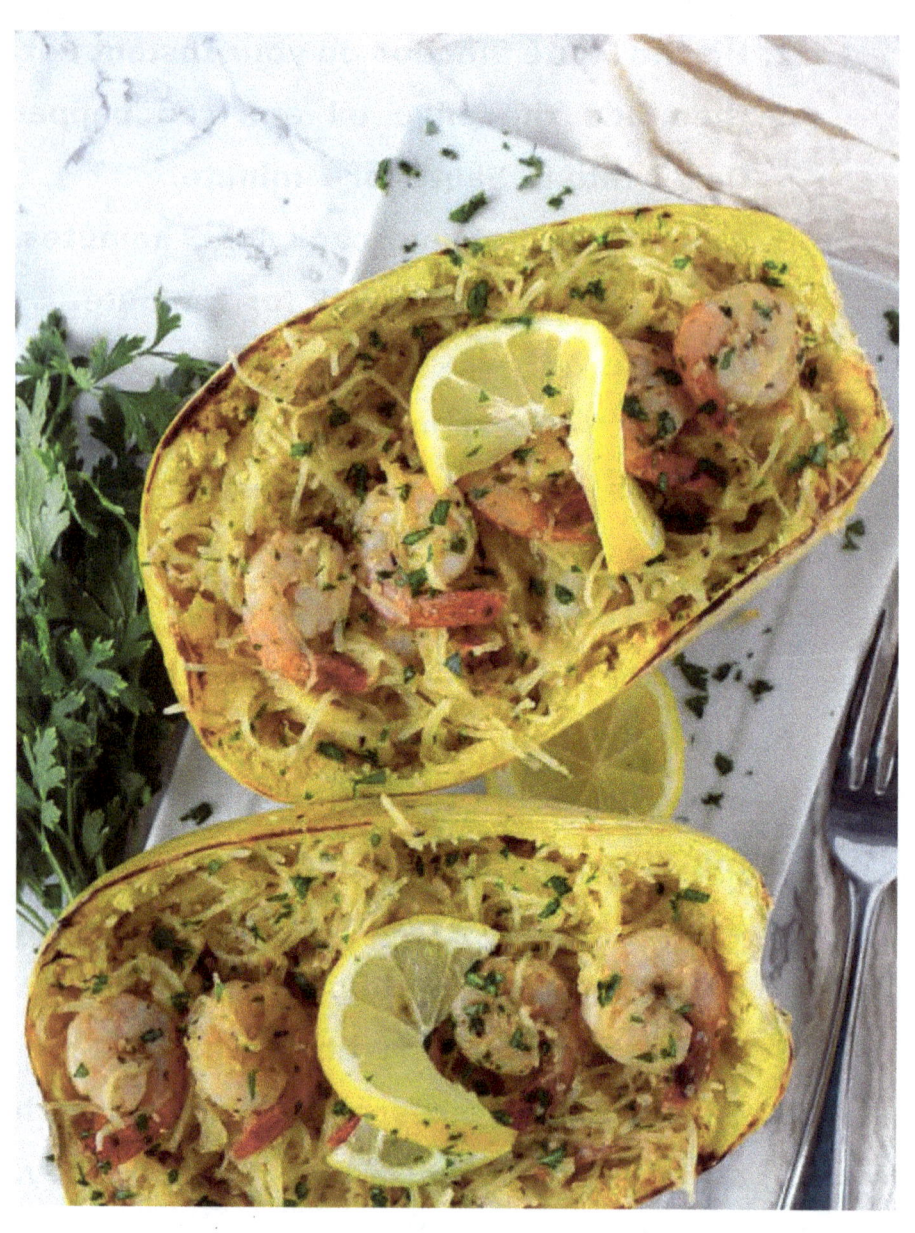

Scallop Teriyaki

Prep time: 5 minutes | Cook time: 5 minutes | Serves 6

2 pounds (907 g) jumbo sea scallops

2 tablespoons olive oil

6 tablespoons pure maple syrup

1 cup coconut aminos

1 teaspoon ground ginger

1 teaspoon garlic powder

1 teaspoon sea salt

1. **Add the olive oil to the Instant pot and heat it on the Sauté settings of your pot.**
2. **Add the scallops to the pot and cook for a minute from each side.**
3. **Stir in all the remaining ingredients in the pot and mix them well.**
4. **Secure the lid and select the Steam function to cook for 3 minutes.**
5. **After the beep, do a Quick release then remove the lid.**
6. **Serve hot.**

Per Serving

calories: 228 | fat: 5.3g | protein: 23.4g | carbs: 21.4g | fiber: 0.5g | sodium: 3664mg

Shrimp and Tomato Creole

Prep time: 20 minutes | Cook time: 7 hours 10 minutes | Serves 4

1 pound (454 g) shrimp (peeled and deveined)
1 tablespoon olive oil
1 (28-ounce / 794-g) can crush whole tomatoes
1 cup celery stalk (sliced)
¾ cup chopped white onion
½ cup green bell pepper (chopped)
1 (8-ounce / 227-g) can tomato sauce
½ teaspoon minced garlic
¼ teaspoon ground black pepper
1 tablespoon Worcestershire sauce
4 drops hot pepper sauce
Salt, to taste
White rice for serving

1. Put the oil to the Instant Pot along with all the ingredients except the shrimp.
2. Secure the cooker lid and keep the pressure handle valve turned to the venting position.
3. Select the Slow Cook function on your cooker and set it on medium heat.

4. Let the mixture cook for 6 hours.
5. Remove the lid afterwards and add the shrimp to the pot.
6. Stir and let the shrimp cook for another 1 hour on Slow Cook function.
7. Keep the lid covered with pressure release handle in the venting position.
8. To serve, pour the juicy shrimp creole over steaming white rice.

Per Serving

calories: 231 | fat: 4.8g | protein: 27.6g | carbs: 23.8g | fiber: 6.1g | sodium: 646mg

Mahi-Mahi and Tomato Bowls

Prep time: 5 minutes | Cook time: 14 minutes | Serves 3

3 (4-ounce / 113-g) mahi-mahi fillets
1½ tablespoons olive oil
½ yellow onion, sliced
½ teaspoon dried oregano
1 tablespoon fresh lemon juice
Salt and freshly ground black pepper, to taste
1 (14-ounce / 397-g) can sugar-free diced tomatoes

1. Add the olive oil to the Instant Pot. Select the Sauté function on it.
2. Add all the ingredient to the pot except the fillets. Cook them for 10 minutes.
3. Press the Cancel key, then add the mahi-mahi fillets to the sauce.
4. Cover the fillets with sauce by using a spoon.
5. Secure the lid and set the Manual function at High Pressure for 4 minutes.

6. **After the beep, do a Quick release then remove the lid.**
7. **Serve the fillets with their sauce, poured on top.**

Per Serving

calories: 265 | fat: 8.6g | protein: 39.1g | carbs: 7.0g | fiber: 3.1g | sodium: 393mg

Alfredo Tuscan Shrimp with Penne

Prep time: 5 minutes | Cook time: 5 minutes | Serves 3

1 pound (454 g) shrimp
1 jar alfredo sauce
1½ cups fresh spinach
1 cup sun-dried tomatoes
1 box penne pasta
1½ teaspoons Tuscan seasoning
3 cups water

1. **Add the water and pasta to a pot over a medium heat, boil until it cooks completely. Then strain the pasta and keep it aside.**
2. **Select the Sauté function on your Instant Pot and add the tomatoes, shrimp, Tuscan seasoning, and alfredo sauce into it.**
3. **Stir and cook until shrimp turn pink in color.**
4. **Now add the spinach leaves to the pot and cook for 5 minutes.**
5. **Add the pasta to the pot and stir well.**
6. **Serve hot.**

Per Serving

calories: 1361 | fat: 70.1g | protein: 55.9g | carbs: 134.4g | fiber: 19.4g | sodium: 933mg

Tuna with Shirataki Noodles

Prep time: 5 minutes | Cook time: 4 minutes | Serves 2

½ can tuna, drained
8 ounces (227 g) Shirataki noodles
½ cup frozen peas
1 (14-ounce / 397-g) can cream mushroom soup
2 ounces (57 g) shredded Cheddar cheese
1½ cups water

1. Add the water with noodles to the base of your Instant Pot.
2. Place the tuna and peas over it. Then pour the mushroom soup on top.
3. Secure the lid and cook with the Manual function at High Pressure for 4 minutes.
4. After the beep, do a Quick release then remove the lid.
5. Stir in shredded cheese to the tuna mix.
6. Serve warm.

Per Serving

calories: 362 | fat: 11.1g | protein: 19.5g | carbs: 46.5g | fiber: 1.5g | sodium: 645mg

Grits with Shrimp

Prep time: 5 minutes | Cook time: 15 minutes | Serves 8

- 1 tablespoon oil
- 2 cups quick grits
- 12 ounces (340 g) Parmesan cheese, shredded
- 2 cups heavy cream
- 24 ounces (680 g) tail-on shrimp
- 2 tablespoons Old Bay seasoning
- A pinch of ground black pepper
- 4 cups water

1. **Add a tablespoon of oil to the Instant Pot. Select the Sauté function for cooking.**
2. **Add the shrimp to the oil and drizzle old bay seasoning over It.**
3. **Cook the shrimp for 3-4 minutes while stirring then set them aside.**
4. **Now add the water, cream, and quick grits to the pot. Select the Manual function for 3 minutes at High Pressure.**
5. **After the beep, do a Quick release then remove the lid.**

6. Add the shredded cheese to the grits then stir well.
7. Take a serving bowl, first pour in the creamy grits mixture then top it with shrimp.
8. Sprinkle black pepper on top then serve hot.

Per Serving

calories: 528 | fat: 38.6g | protein: 30.7g | carbs: 15.2g | fiber: 0.7g | sodium: 1249mg

Basil Pesto

Prep time: 5 minutes | Cook time: 0 minutes | Makes 1 cup

2 cups packed fresh basil leaves
3 garlic cloves, peeled
½ cup freshly grated Parmesan cheese
½ cup extra-virgin olive oil
¼ cup pine nuts
Kosher salt and freshly ground black pepper, to taste

1. Place all the ingredients, except for the salt and pepper, in a food processor. Pulse a few times until smoothly puréed. Season with salt and pepper to taste.
2. Store in an airtight container in the fridge for up to 2 weeks.

Per Serving

calories: 100 | fat: 10.2g | protein: 2.2g | carbs: 1.2g | fiber: 0g | sodium: 72mg

Orange-Garlic Dressing

Prep time: 5 minutes | Cook time: 0 minutes | Serves 2

¼ cup extra-virgin olive oil

1 orange, zested

2 tablespoons freshly squeezed orange juice

¾ teaspoon za'atar seasoning

1 teaspoon garlic powder

½ teaspoon salt

¼ teaspoon Dijon mustard

Freshly ground black pepper, to taste

1. Whisk together all ingredients in a bowl until well combined.
2. Serve immediately or refrigerate until ready to serve.

Per Serving

calories: 287 | fat: 26.7g | protein: 1.2g | carbs: 12.0g | fiber: 2.1g | sodium: 592mg

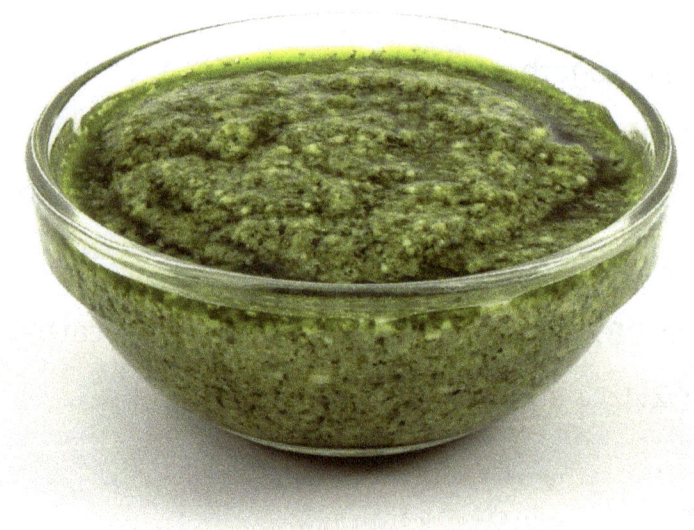

Creamy Cider Yogurt Dressing

Prep time: 5 minutes | Cook time: 0 minutes | Serves 2

1 cup plain, unsweetened, full-fat Greek yogurt

½ cup extra-virgin olive oil

½ lemon, juiced

1 tablespoon chopped fresh oregano

1 tablespoon apple cider vinegar

½ teaspoon dried parsley

½ teaspoon kosher salt

¼ teaspoon garlic powder

¼ teaspoon freshly ground black pepper

1. **In a large bowl, whisk all ingredients to combine.**
2. **Serve chilled or at room temperature.**

Per Serving

calories: 407 | fat: 40.7g | protein: 8.3g | carbs: 3.8g | fiber: 0.5g | sodium: 382mg

Basic French Vinaigrette

Prep time: 5 minutes | Cook time: 0 minutes | Serves 2

- 3 tablespoons apple cider vinegar
- 2 tablespoons minced shallot (or 1 tablespoon minced red onion)
- 1 tablespoon balsamic vinegar
- ½ teaspoon dried thyme
- 1 teaspoon Dijon mustard
- ¼ cup olive oil
- Salt and black pepper, to taste

1. **Stir together the apple cider vinegar, shallot, and balsamic vinegar in a medium jar with a tight-fitting lid. Allow to sit for 5 minutes.**
2. **Stir in the mustard and thyme. Whisk in the olive oil in a slow, steady stream and season to taste with salt and pepper.**
3. **Store in an airtight container in the fridge for up to 5 days.**

Per Serving

calories: 256 | fat: 27.1g | protein: 0.3g | carbs: 3.4g | fiber: 0.4g | sodium: 207mg

Mediterranean Lamb Bowl

Preparation Time: 15 minutes

Cooking Time: 15 minutes

Servings: 2

Ingredients:

- 2 tablespoons extra-virgin olive oil
- ¼ cup diced yellow onion
- 1 pound ground lamb
- 1 teaspoon dried mint
- 1 teaspoon dried parsley
- ½ teaspoon red pepper flakes
- ¼ teaspoon garlic powder
- 1 cup cooked rice
- ½ teaspoon za'atar seasoning
- ½ cup halved cherry tomatoes
- 1 cucumber, peeled and diced
- 1 cup store-bought hummus or Garlic-Lemon Hummus
- 1 cup crumbled feta cheese
- 2 pita breads, warmed (optional)

Directions:

1. In a large sauté pan or skillet, heat the olive oil over medium heat and cook the onion for about 2 minutes, until fragrant.
2. Add the lamb and mix well, breaking up the meat as you cook. Once the lamb is halfway cooked, add mint, parsley, red pepper flakes, and garlic powder.
3. In a medium bowl, mix together the cooked rice and za'atar, then divide between individual serving bowls. Add the seasoned lamb, then top the bowls with the tomatoes, cucumber, hummus, feta, and pita (if using).

Nutrition:

Calories: 1,312; Protein: 62g; Carbohydrates: 62g; Fat: 96g

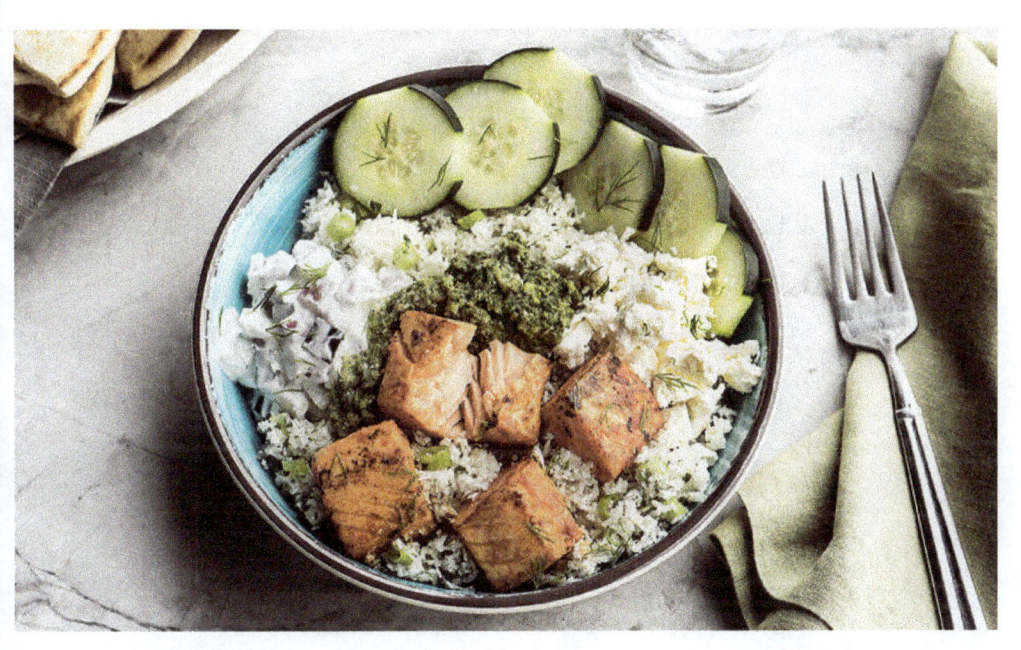

Lamb Burger

Preparation Time: 15 minutes

Cooking Time: 15 minutes

Servings: 4

Ingredients:

- 1 pound ground lamb
- ½ small red onion, grated
- 1 tablespoon dried parsley
- 1 teaspoon dried oregano
- 1 teaspoon ground cumin
- 1 teaspoon garlic powder
- ½ teaspoon dried mint
- ¼ teaspoon paprika
- ¼ teaspoon kosher salt
- 1/8 teaspoon freshly ground black pepper
- Extra-virgin olive oil, for panfrying
- 4 pita breads, for serving (optional)
- Tzatziki Sauce, for serving (optional)
- Pickled Onions, for serving (optional)

Directions:

1. In a bowl, combine the lamb, onion, parsley, oregano, cumin, garlic powder, mint, paprika, salt,

and pepper. Divide the meat into 4 small balls and work into smooth discs.

2. In a large sauté pan or skillet, heat a drizzle of olive oil over medium heat or brush a grill with oil and set it too medium.

3. Cook the patties for 4 to 5 minutes on each side, until cooked through and juices run clear. Enjoy lamb burgers in pitas, topped with tzatziki sauce and pickled onions (if using).

Nutrition:

Calories: 328 ; Protein: 19g ; Carbohydrates: 2g ; Fat: 27g

Quick Herbed Lamb and Pasta

Preparation Time: 15 minutes

Cooking Time: 15 minutes

Servings: 4

Ingredients:

- 3 thick lamb sausages, removed from casing and crumbled
- 1 medium shallot, chopped
- 1½ cups diced baby portobello mushrooms
- 1 teaspoon garlic powder
- 1 tablespoon extra-virgin olive oil
- 1 pound bean-based penne pasta
- 4 medium Roma tomatoes, chopped
- 1 (14.5-ounce) can crushed tomatoes
- 3 tablespoons heavy cream

Directions:

1. Heat a large sauté pan or skillet over medium-high heat. Add the sausage to the skillet and cook for about 5 minutes, mixing and breaking the sausage up until the sausage is halfway cooked.
2. Reduce the heat to medium-low and add the shallot. Continue cooking for about 3 minutes, until they're soft.

3. Add the mushrooms, garlic powder, and olive oil and cook for 5 to 7 minutes, until the mushrooms have reduced in size by half and all the water is cooked out.
4. Meanwhile, bring a large pot of water to a boil and cook the pasta according to the package directions, until al dente. Drain and set aside.
5. To the skillet, add the chopped and canned tomatoes and cook for 7 to 10 minutes, until the liquid thickens slightly.
6. Reduce the heat and add the cream, mixing well. Plate the pasta first and top with the sausage mixture.

Nutrition:

Calories: 706, Protein: 45g, Carbohydrates: 79g, Fat: 31g

Marinated Lamb Kebabs with Crunchy Yogurt Dressing

Preparation Time: 15 minutes

Cooking Time: 15 minutes

Servings: 4

Ingredients:

- ½ cup plain, unsweetened, full-fat Greek yogurt
- ¼ cup extra-virgin olive oil
- ¼ cup freshly squeezed lemon juice
- 1 teaspoon grated lemon zest
- 2 garlic cloves, minced
- 2 tablespoons honey
- 2 tablespoons balsamic vinegar
- 1½ teaspoons oregano, fresh, minced
- 1 teaspoon thyme, fresh, minced
- 1 bay leaf
- 1 teaspoon kosher salt
- ½ teaspoon freshly ground black pepper
- ½ teaspoon red pepper flakes
- 2 pounds leg of lamb, trimmed, cleaned and cut into 1-inch pieces

- 1 large red onion, diced large
- 1 recipe Crunchy Yogurt Dip
- Parsley, chopped, for garnish
- Lemon wedges, for garnish

Directions:

1. In a bowl or large resealable bag, combine the yogurt, olive oil, lemon juice and zest, garlic, honey, balsamic vinegar, oregano, thyme, bay leaf, salt, pepper, and red pepper flakes. Mix well.
2. Add the lamb pieces and marinate, refrigerated, for 30 minutes. Preheat the oven to 375°F. Thread the lamb onto the skewers, alternating with chunks of red onion as desired.
3. Put the skewers onto a baking sheet and roast for 10 to 15 minutes, rotating every 5 minutes to ensure that they cook evenly.
4. Plate the skewers and allow them to rest briefly. Top or serve with the yogurt dressing. To finish, garnish with fresh chopped parsley and a lemon wedge.

Nutrition:

Calories: 578 ; Protein: 56g ; Carbohydrates: 20g ; Fat: 30g

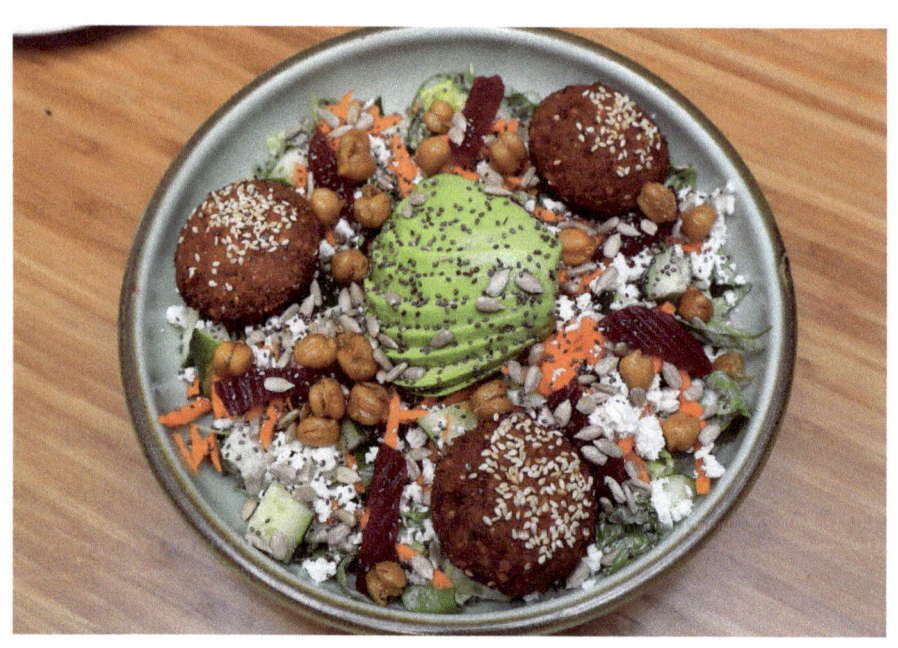

Garlic Pork Tenderloin and Lemony Orzo

Preparation Time: 15 minutes

Cooking Time: 20 minutes

Servings: 6

Ingredients:

- 1 pound pork tenderloin
- ½ teaspoon Shawarma Spice Rub
- 1 tablespoon salt
- ½ teaspoon coarsely ground black pepper
- ½ teaspoon garlic powder
- 6 tablespoons extra-virgin olive oil
- 3 cups Lemony Orzo

Directions:

1. Preheat the oven to 350°F. Rub the pork with shawarma seasoning, salt, pepper, and garlic powder and drizzle with the olive oil.
2. Put the pork on a baking sheet and roast for 20 minutes, or until desired doneness. Remove the pork from the oven and let rest for 10 minutes. Assemble the pork on a plate with the orzo and enjoy.

Nutrition:

Calories: 579

Protein: 33g

Carbohydrates: 37g

Fat: 34g

Roasted Pork with Apple-Dijon Sauce

Preparation Time: 15 minutes

Cooking Time: 40 minutes

Servings: 8

Ingredients:

- 1½ tablespoons extra-virgin olive oil
- 1 (12-ounce) pork tenderloin
- ¼ teaspoon kosher salt
- ¼ teaspoon freshly ground black pepper
- ¼ cup apple jelly
- ¼ cup apple juice
- 2 to 3 tablespoons Dijon mustard
- ½ tablespoon cornstarch
- ½ tablespoon cream

Directions:

1. Preheat the oven to 325°F. In a large sauté pan or skillet, heat the olive oil over medium heat.
2. Add the pork to the skillet, using tongs to turn and sear the pork on all sides. Once seared, sprinkle pork with salt and pepper, and set it on a small baking sheet.

3. In the same skillet, with the juices from the pork, mix the apple jelly, juice, and mustard into the pan juices. Heat thoroughly over low heat, stirring consistently for 5 minutes. Spoon over the pork.
4. Put the pork in the oven and roast for 15 to 17 minutes, or 20 minutes per pound. Every 10 to 15 minutes, baste the pork with the apple-mustard sauce.
5. Once the pork tenderloin is done, remove it from the oven and let it rest for 15 minutes. Then, cut it into 1-inch slices.
6. In a small pot, blend the cornstarch with cream. Heat over low heat. Add the pan juices into the pot, stirring for 2 minutes, until thickened. Serve the sauce over the pork.

Nutrition:

Calories: 146; Protein: 13g; Carbohydrates: 8g; Fat: 7g

Pressure Cooker Moroccan Pot Roast

Preparation Time: 15 minutes

Cooking Time: 50 minutes

Servings: 4

Ingredients:

- 8 ounces mushrooms, sliced
- 4 tablespoons extra-virgin olive oil
- 3 small onions, cut into 2-inch pieces
- 2 tablespoons paprika
- 1½ tablespoons garam masala
- 2 teaspoons salt
- ¼ teaspoon ground white pepper
- 2 tablespoons tomato paste
- 1 small eggplant, peeled and diced
- 1¼ cups low-sodium beef broth
- ½ cup halved apricots
- 1/3 cup golden raisins
- 3 pounds beef chuck roast
- 2 tablespoons honey
- 1 tablespoon dried mint
- 2 cups cooked brown rice

Directions:

1. Set an electric pressure cooker to Sauté and put the mushrooms and oil in the cooker. Sauté for 5 minutes, then add the onions, paprika, garam masala, salt, and white pepper. Stir in the tomato paste and continue to sauté.
2. Add the eggplant and sauté for 5 more minutes, until softened. Pour in the broth. Add the apricots and raisins. Sear the meat for 2 minutes on each side. Close and lock the lid and set the pressure cooker too high for 50 minutes.
3. When cooking is complete, quick release the pressure. Carefully remove the lid, then remove the meat from the sauce and break it into pieces. While the meat is removed, stir honey and mint into the sauce.
4. Assemble plates with ½ cup of brown rice, ½ cup of pot roast sauce, and 3 to 5 pieces of pot roast.

Nutrition:

Calories: 829 ; Protein: 69g; Carbohydrates: 70g; Fat: 34g

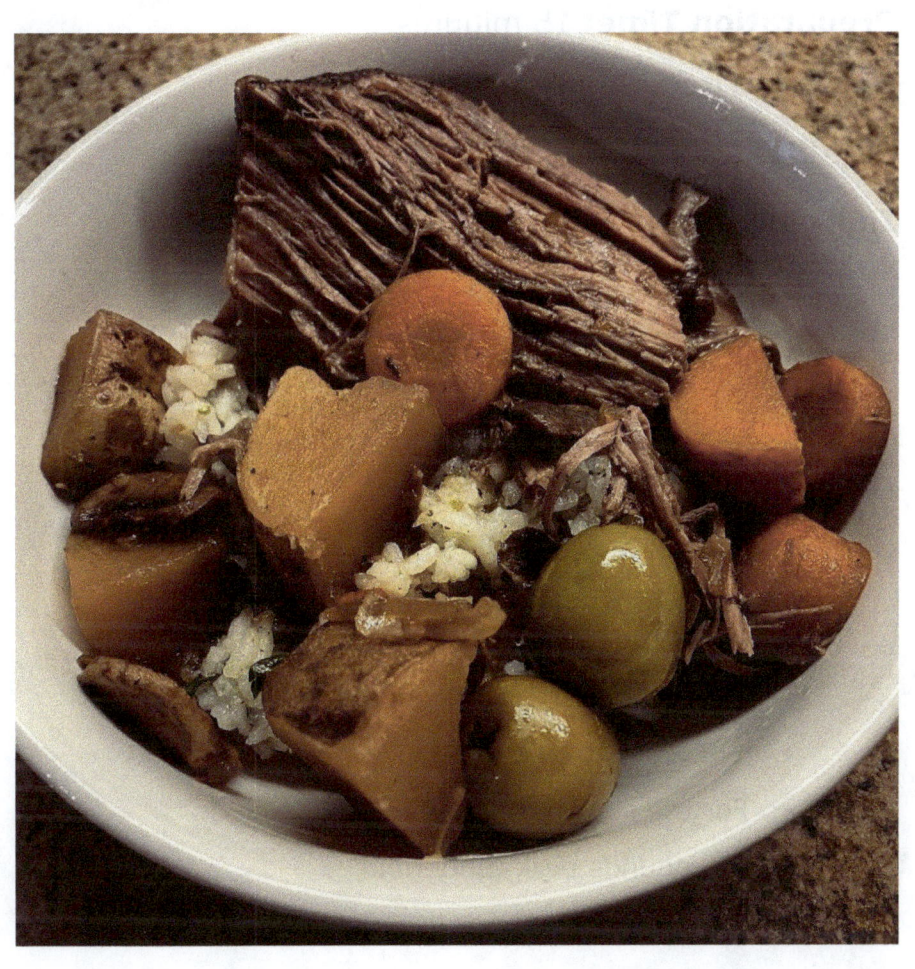

Shawarma Pork Tenderloin with Pitas

Preparation Time: 15 minutes
Cooking Time: 35 minutes
Servings: 8

Ingredients:

- For the shawarma spice rub:
- 1 teaspoon ground cumin
- 1 teaspoon ground coriander
- 1 teaspoon ground turmeric
- ¾ teaspoon sweet Spanish paprika
- ½ teaspoon ground cloves
- ¼ teaspoon salt
- ¼ teaspoon freshly ground black pepper
- 1/8 teaspoon ground cinnamon
- For the shawarma:
- 1½ pounds pork tenderloin
- 3 tablespoons extra-virgin olive oil
- 1 tablespoon garlic powder
- Salt
- Freshly ground black pepper
- 1½ tablespoons Shawarma Spice Rub
- 4 pita pockets, halved, for serving

- 1 to 2 tomatoes, sliced, for serving
- ¼ cup Pickled Onions, for serving
- ¼ cup Pickled Turnips, for serving
- ¼ cup store-bought hummus or Garlic-Lemon Hummus

Directions:

1. To Make the Shawarma Seasoning:
2. In a small bowl, combine the cumin, coriander, turmeric, paprika, cloves, salt, pepper, and cinnamon and set aside.
3. To Make the Shawarma:
4. Preheat the oven to 400°F. Put the pork tenderloin on a plate and cover with olive oil and garlic powder on each side.
5. Season with salt and pepper and rub each side of the tenderloin with a generous amount of shawarma spices.
6. Place the pork tenderloin in the center of a roasting pan and roast for 20 minutes per pound, or until the meat begins to bounce back as you poke it.
7. If it feels like there's still fluid under the skin, continue cooking. Check every 5 to 7 minutes until it reaches the desired tenderness and juices run clear.

8. Remove the pork from the oven and let rest for 10 minutes. Serve the pork tenderloin shawarma with pita pockets, tomatoes, Pickled Onions (if using), Pickled Turnips (if using), and hummus.

Nutrition:

Calories: 316

Protein: 29g

Carbohydrates: 17g

Fat: 15g

Desserts

Honey Almonds

Preparation Time: 10 minutes

Cooking Time: 0 minutes

Servings: 2

Ingredients:

- 1 Tablespoon Rosemary, Fresh & Minced
- 1 Cup Almonds, Raw & Whole
- 1 Tablespoon Honey, Raw
- ¼ Teaspoon Sea Salt, Fine
- Nonstick Cooking Spray

Directions:

1. Get out a skillet and heat it up over medium heat. In this skillet you'll combine your salt, almonds and rosemary. Mix well. You'll need to cook for a full minute and stir frequently.
2. Drizzle your honey in and cook for another four minutes while stirring frequently. Your almonds should start to darken near the edges and be well coated.
3. Remove your almonds from heat, and spread them onto a pan that's been coated with nonstick cooking

spray. They should cool for ten minutes, and then you can break them apart before serving.

Nutrition:

Calories: 149; Protein: 5 Grams; Fat: 12 Grams; Carbs: 8 Grams; Sodium: 78 mg

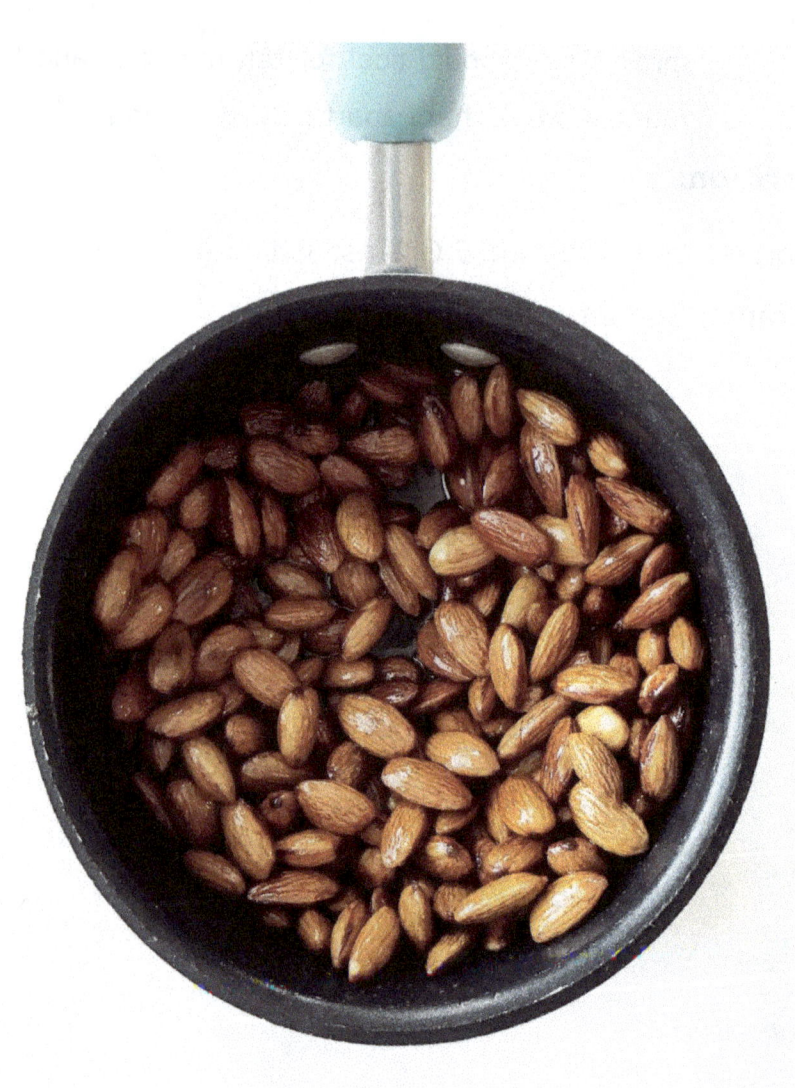

Chocolate-Dipped Citrus Fruit

Preparation Time: 15 minutes, plus 15 minutes to chill

Cooking Time: 5 minutes

Servings: 2

Ingredients:

- 4 ounces 60% dark chocolate, broken into pieces
- 1 tablespoon coconut oil
- 3 clementine, peeled and segmented
- 1 navel orange, peeled and segmented
- 3 mandarin oranges, peeled and segmented

Directions:

1. Line a baking sheet with parchment paper.
2. In a small saucepan, bring about a cup of water to a boil, then reduce heat to a simmer. Place a heat-proof medium bowl on top of the saucepan to make a double boiler. Add the chocolate and coconut oil, and stir gently with a wooden spoon until the mixture is smooth, about 5 minutes.
3. One at a time, dip the tip of each citrus segment into the melted chocolate, and place onto the prepared baking sheet, leaving about ½ inch between pieces.
4. Place in the refrigerator to set, about 15 minutes.

Nutrition:

Calories: 92; Total Fat: 5g; Saturated Fat: 3g; Protein 1g; Carbohydrates: 11g; Fiber: 2g; Sodium: 1mg

Banana-Cinnamon "Ice Cream"

Preparation Time: 10 minutes

Cooking Time: 0 minutes

Servings: 2

Ingredients:

- 4 medium frozen bananas, cut into 2-inch chunks
- ¼ cup 100% maple syrup
- 1 teaspoon ground cinnamon

Directions:

1. Allow the frozen banana chunks to rest at room temperature for 5 minutes, then place in a food processor or blender.
2. Add the maple syrup and cinnamon, and purée until well combined.
3. Serve immediately, or store in a freezer-safe container in the freezer until later.

Nutrition:

Calories: 159; Total Fat: 0g; Saturated Fat: 0g; Protein: 1g; Carbohydrates: 41 g; Fiber: 3g; Sodium: 4mg

Sweet Peach Jam

Preparation Time: 10 minutes

Cooking Time: 16 minutes

Servings: 20

Ingredients:

- 1 1/2 lb. fresh peaches, pitted and chopped
- 1/2 tbsp vanilla
- 1/4 cup maple syrup

Directions:

1. Put all of the ingredients in the air fryer and stir well.
2. Seal pot and cook on high for 1 minute.
3. Once done, allow to release pressure naturally. Remove lid.
4. Set pot on sauté mode and cook for 15 minutes or until jam thickened.
5. Pour into the container and store it in the fridge.

Nutrition:

Calories – 16

Protein – 0.1 g.

Fat – 0 g.

Carbs – 3.7 g.

Pear Sauce

Preparation Time: 10 minutes

Cooking Time: 15 minutes

Servings: 6

Ingredients:

- 10 pears, sliced
- 1 cup apple juice
- 1 1/2 tsp cinnamon
- 1/4 tsp nutmeg

Directions:

1. Put all of the ingredients in the air fryer and stir well.
2. Seal pot and cook on high for 15 minutes.
3. Once done, allow to release pressure naturally for 10 minutes then release remaining using quick release. Remove lid.
4. Blend the pear mixture using an immersion blender until smooth.
5. Serve and enjoy.

Nutrition:

Calories – 222

Protein – 1.3 g.

Fat – 0.6 g.

Carbs – 58.2 g.

Brownie Muffins

Preparation Time: 10 minutes

Cooking Time: 10 minutes

Servings: 12

Ingredients:

- 1 package Betty Crocker fudge brownie mix
- ¼ cup walnuts, chopped
- 1 egg
- 1/3 cup vegetable oil
- 2 teaspoons water

Directions:

1. Grease 12 muffin molds. Set aside.
2. In a bowl, put all ingredients together.
3. Place the mixture into the prepared muffin molds.
4. Press "Power Button" of Air Fry Oven and turn the dial to select the "Air Fry" mode.
5. Press the Time button and again turn the dial to set the cooking time to 10 minutes.
6. Now push the Temp button and rotate the dial to set the temperature at 300 degrees F.
7. Press "Start/Pause" button to start.
8. When the unit beeps to show that it is preheated, open the lid.

9. Arrange the muffin molds in "Air Fry Basket" and insert in the oven.
10. **Place the muffin molds onto a wire rack to cool for about 10 minutes.**
11. **Carefully, invert the muffins onto the wire rack to completely cool before serving.**

Nutrition:

Calories – 168

Protein – 2 g.

Fat – 8.9 g.

Carbs – 20.8 g.

French Toast Bites

Preparation Time: 5 minutes

Cooking Time: 15 minutes

Servings: 8

Ingredients:

- Almond milk
- Cinnamon
- Sweetener
- 3 eggs
- 4 pieces wheat bread

Directions:

1. Preheat the air fryer oven to 360 degrees.
2. Whisk eggs and thin out with almond milk.
3. Mix 1/3 cup of sweetener with lots of cinnamon.
4. Tear bread in half, ball up pieces and press together to form a ball.
5. Soak bread balls in egg and then roll into cinnamon sugar, making sure to thoroughly coat.
6. Place coated bread balls into the air fryer oven and bake 15 minutes.

Nutrition:

Calories – 289; Protein – 0 g; Fat – 11 g; Carbs – 17 g.

Cinnamon Sugar Roasted Chickpeas

Preparation Time: 5 minutes

Cooking Time: 10 minutes

Servings: 2

Ingredients:

- 1 tbsp. sweetener
- 1 tbsp. cinnamon
- 1 C. chickpeas

Directions:

1. Preheat air fryer oven to 390 degrees.
2. Rinse and drain chickpeas.
3. Mix all ingredients together and add to air fryer.
4. Pour into the Oven rack/basket. Place the Rack on the middle-shelf of the Air fryer oven. Set temperature to 390°F, and set time to 10 minutes.

Nutrition:

Calories – 111

Protein – 16 g.

Fat – 19 g.

Carbs – 18 g.

Glazed Pears with Hazelnuts

Prep time: 10 minutes | Cook time: 20 minutes | Serves 4

4 pears, peeled, cored, and quartered lengthwise

1 cup apple juice

1 tablespoon grated fresh ginger

½ cup pure maple syrup

¼ cup chopped hazelnuts

1. **Put the pears in a pot, then pour in the apple juice. Bring to a boil over medium-high heat, then reduce the heat to medium-low. Stir constantly.**
2. **Cover and simmer for an additional 15 minutes or until the pears are tender.**
3. **Meanwhile, combine the ginger and maple syrup in a saucepan. Bring to a boil over medium-high heat. Stir frequently. Turn off the heat and transfer the syrup to a small bowl and let sit until ready to use.**

4. **Transfer the pears in a large serving bowl with a slotted spoon, then top the pears with syrup.**
5. **Spread the hazelnuts over the pears and serve immediately.**

Per Serving

calories: 287 | fat: 3.1g | protein: 2.2g | carbs: 66.9g | fiber: 7.0g | sodium: 8mg

Lemony Blackberry Granita

Prep time: 10 minutes | Cook time: 0 minutes | Serves 4

1 pound (454 g) fresh blackberries

½ cup raw honey

1 teaspoon chopped fresh thyme

½ cup water

¼ cup freshly squeezed lemon juice

1. **Put all the ingredients in a food processor, then pulse to purée.**
2. **Pour the mixture through a sieve into a baking dish. Discard the seeds remain in the sieve.**
3. **Put the baking dish in the freezer for 2 hours. Remove the dish from the refrigerator and stir to break any frozen parts.**
4. **Return the dish back to the freezer for an hour, then stir to break any frozen parts again.**
5. **Return the dish to the freezer for 4 hours until the granita is completely frozen.**

6. Remove it from the freezer and mash to serve.

Per Serving

calories: 183 | fat: 1.1g | protein: 2.2g | carbs: 45.9g | fiber: 6.0g | sodium: 6mg

www.ingramcontent.com/pod-product-compliance
Lightning Source LLC
Chambersburg PA
CBHW070734030426
42336CB00013B/1974